How to develop real human superpowers

I0447731

HTeBooks

Disclaimer

This book is designed to provide condensed information. It is not intended to reprint all the information that is otherwise available, but instead to complement, amplify and supplement other texts. You are urged to read all the available material, learn as much as possible and tailor the information to your individual needs.

Every effort has been made to make this book as complete and as accurate as possible. However, there may be mistakes, both typographical and in content. Therefore, this text should be used only as a general guide and not as the ultimate source of information. The purpose of this book is to educate.

The author or the publisher shall have neither liability nor responsibility to any person or entity regarding any loss or damage caused, or alleged to have been caused, directly or indirectly, by the information contained in this book.

Table of Contents

Real Human SuperPowers?

Echolocation, impressive feats of strength? Although seemingly impossible, there are people who already have these abilities, which they acquired through diligent study and years of training.

The human mind is an incredible thing. It can adapt to environmental and physical changes. In extreme cases when the body is subjected to horrific living conditions or accidents, the brain rewires everything at cellular level – a form of micro evolution or mutation born out of need. This allows the physical self to function, or at least, survive. Once the body is out of presumed danger, the brain rewires again in an effort to "normalize" living conditions. In many cases, this form of micro evolution or reinvention becomes a continuous life-long process.

This condition is called **neuroplasticity**, and it can be seen when:

*)A visually-impaired person uses echolocation to map his surroundings.

*)A child born with spinal muscular atrophy acquires bulk and mass by the age of 18, only by sheer willpower.

Neuroplasticity can also be harnessed to improve mental well-being, and to push the body into performing incredible and uncommon feats of endurance and strength.

Like all things worth investing in, rewiring the brain takes time and practice. But the benefits after mastering this skill are beyond incredible.

This book contains information on how to unlock your unique powers through study and training. You can acquire super human powers without subjecting yourself to dangerous experimentations, or casting magic spells, or spending lots of money on technology and weaponry.

Aside from relying on neuroplasticity, this book also has specific recommendations for both mental and physical exercises that can be used to hone your "powers" faster.

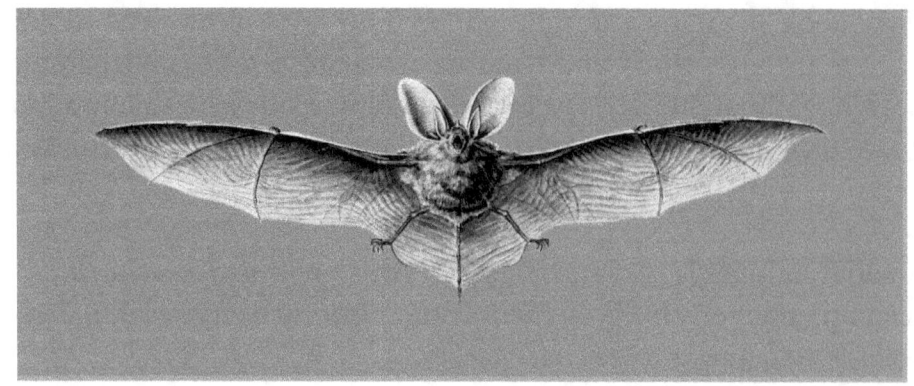

Fruit bats have large ears, which allow them to hear well in near or total darkness. Nocturnal by nature, these bats use echolocation to forage for food and avoid predators.
Image source: www.pixabay.com

Echolocation (a.k.a. bio sonar)

Numerous animals use echolocation to navigate through their world. They emit calls and use corresponding echoes to discern sound frequencies as these bounce off objects. Frequency strength denotes distance, size, and speed. Animals use this skill for foraging, hunting, mating, migrating, nesting, and even escaping danger.

Fruit bats and flying foxes are known for their echolocation skills, but other animals like: *odontocetes* (e.g. beaked whales, dolphins, porpoises, and sperm whales,) cave dwelling birds (.e.g. swifts and oilbirds,) and earth burrowers (e.g. moles and shrews) also use sound waves to find what they need in near or total darkness. These animals produce more than 200 clicks per second when they are hunting or when they sense danger nearby.

Human echolocation.

Some people who lost their sight at an early age have learned to use sound frequency to map their surroundings (a.k.a. acoustic way finding, auditory mapping, or flash sonar.)
This gives them more mobility, and heightens their other senses. Sighted people who live or work in darkness (e.g. spelunkers, sewer workers, etc.) use echolocation skills when navigating dangerous areas.

How Does Human Echolocation Work?
It begins with sonar emission: a unique sound or noise coming from the host. This can be done by calling, clicking, or humming. Others snap their fingers, or tap their walking sticks/tools on any hard surface. Shuffling or stomp their feet works too. Sonar emission should be easy to produce, easy to control, and can be repeated without any hardship to the host. This should be just loud enough for sound frequency to travel a short distance away, but won't drown out other auditory stimuli, especially returning resonances or echoes.

The host then listens for echoes that bounce off nearby objects. Differences in time delays denote composition (e.g. fabric, wood, or metal,) gaps in between, and direction or speed of moving objects.
Using both ears, the host compares the volume of returning sounds. If these ring louder in the right ear, then the brain logically assumes that the source is nearer to the right side. The body involuntarily moves in the same direction. This is called sound perception.

Some people claim that they can feel returning sounds on their faces, describing the sensation as similar "to the passing of gentle air currents." The natural tendency is to move their faces (rather than the entire body) to acquire better "reception." This is called facial mapping, or perceiving facial pressure.

MRI or magnetic resonance imaging results show that people who regularly practice sound perception have hyperactive cortical areas, specifically within the parietal lobe (middle part of the brain.) These areas are apparently devoted solely to echo processing. The same is true for those who practice facial mapping, but they experience hyperactivity in the cerebrum (front part of the brain) too, which is responsible for the sense of touch.

Learning echolocation takes years of practice. But an hour or more of daily intense training yields notable results.

Advantages of human echolocation
For visually-impaired people, this skill provides mobility and independence. Instead of relying on a sighted person or on a seeing-eye dog, echolocation allows them to ride bikes, run marathons, and explore unfamiliar areas/terrains all on their own. This skill heightens their *audioception* (sense of hearing) considerably, and improves their *olfacoception* (sense of smell,) and *tactioception* (sense of touch) too. Some report that their gustaoception (sense of taste) becomes more refined.

For sighted people, practicing echolocation allows them to move in darkness without the aid of artificial light. This dramatically increases night vision acuity, and helps heighten the remaining senses as well.

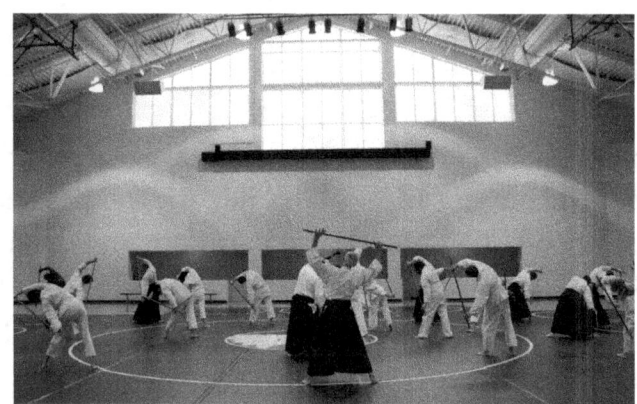

One of the guiding philosophies of Aikido (Japanese martial art)
is to study the energy coming from the environment. This entails listening well,

and sometimes making flash decisions solely from auditory stimuli.
Image source: www.pixabay.com

A number of studies suggests that martial arts practitioners who regularly use echolocation during training have faster reflexes, and think/react better in potentially dangerous situations.

Basic Guidelines on Echolocation Training

Have an EENT (eye, ear, nose, and throat) doctor check your hearing.

Echolocation entails good hearing – or at least, a pair of working auditory canals that can gather as much sound as possible. Have your doctor check for any existing or recent damage to the outer ear (specifically the ear canal and eardrum,) middle ear (malleus and stapes,) and inner ear (cochlea and the nerves nearest the brain.)

Having any ear-related ailment can prevent you from honing your echolocation skills. These include:

- AIED or autoimmune inner ear disease (inflammatory condition that afflicts the inner ear)
- Barotrauma (ear injury caused by abrupt changes in air/water pressure)
- *Cerumen* impaction (excessive and immovable earwax buildup on the ear canals)
- Growth of cysts or tumors in inner or middle ear
- Ménière's disease (affects inner ear and vestibular system)
- *Otitis media* (infection of the middle ear) and *otitis externa* (infection of the outer ear)
- *Otosclerosis* (abnormal buildup of bone or tissue in middle ear)
- Perforated eardrum (ruptured eardrums) and
- Tinnitus (persistent and/or chronic noises due to damaged ear nerves)

Only when your doctor gives you a clean bill of health can you start your echolocation training. And part of that training is learning how to take care, and how to safely clean your ears.

- Clean your ears daily. When you shower or wash your face, gently soap and scrub the fleshy part of your ears, too. Take care not to push water or soap into the ear canal. Gently rinse and dry off.

- If you have never really cleaned you ear canals before, and you are currently suffering from one or more symptoms of *cerumen* impaction, like: chronic ache in the affected ear, fullness or impaired hearing, or a mild cheese-like odor coming out from affected ear, it is best to ask your doctor to remove blockages for you. Don't attempt this on your own, or you can permanently damage your middle ear.
- Always lower down the volume of the devices you are using, (e.g. radio, TV, phones, etc.). Listening to extremely loud music, or chronically subjecting your hearing to noises louder than 80 decibels a minute destroys hair cells *(cilia)* in the cochlea. Mild to moderate damage causes tinnitus, but complete destruction means progressive/permanent hearing loss.
- Wear any kind of hearing protection whenever possible. These include: ear muffs, foam earplugs, noise cancelling headphones, *otoplastics*, silicon plugs, and wax balls.

Meditate. Pay attention to minute details.

Part of echolocation training is learning to differentiate between sounds. This can be achieved by closing your eyes, sitting quietly (so as not to make any sound emissions,) and making mental notes on what objects yield specific reverberations. This is **auditory meditation**, which is an intense form of listening.

Learn common ambient noises by heart. These may include: low hum of a nearby machine, rustling of tree leaves on branches, and scraping footsteps on concrete sidewalks.

What do ordinary days or nights sound like in your room, house, or town?
How do these change when something uncommon happens?

Learn to differentiate between seemingly same sounds from same sources. For example: a silver coin dropped on a wooden table makes a different sound when you drop the same piece on a marble, metal, or fabric-lined surface. The height from which the coin is dropped alters sound. Different people dropping the same coin on the same surface from the same height likewise affects resonance quality. In fact, you can produce two different sounds by simply switching hands, or produce a series of different reverberations when you pick up and drop same coin in quick successions.

It is recommended that you practice auditory meditation at least 30 minutes per day for the first 2 weeks. Prolong your meditation period to an hour afterwards. Choose any safe area where you can sit or rest undisturbed. It doesn't matter if you are in your room, or in the library, or outdoors. What's important is that you can still and just listen. Pay attention to the smallest sounds around you.

Make your own unique sound emission.

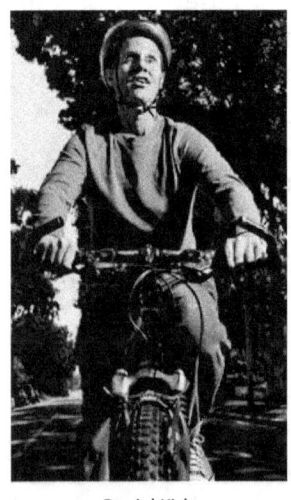

Daniel Kish.
Image source:
www.techly.com.au/daniel-kish

Daniel Kish is the President of World Access to the Blind. He lost his vision when he was only 13 months old. He uses echolocation to ride his bicycle, hike through mountain trails, and travel to different countries on his own. He is an accomplished cook, an avid swimmer, and an enthusiastic dancer.

He makes his own unique sound emissions by clicking using his tongue. He produces a series of loud, mechanical-sounding clicks, and then listens as the sound bounces off objects around him. He calls this his "flash sonar."

Vocal sound emissions, like Kish's, allow you to create sound waves without using your hands or specialized tools. These are the hardest to maintain though, because many elements can go wrong (e.g. voice faltering midway, sound weakening.)

Consistency is essential when making echo-producing sound emissions.

9

If you are clicking, humming or even whistling, you need to use the same duration, intensity, pitch, and timbre all the time. Otherwise, echoes become lost in background noises.

You can opt for finger snapping or even tapping surfaces with your fingers or nails. Shuffling your feet, tapping your shoe, or knocking sticks (or any object) on walls or floors are good too. These are easier to reproduce, but may limit your use of hands or feet, or overall mobility.

The best sound emissions to use are the ones that come naturally to you, and don't become tiresome during prolonged repetition.

It is recommended that you practice making your sound emissions for at least 10 to 20 minutes every day, until you can make these as consistent as possible.

Study echoes. Find your own unique way of gathering auditory information.

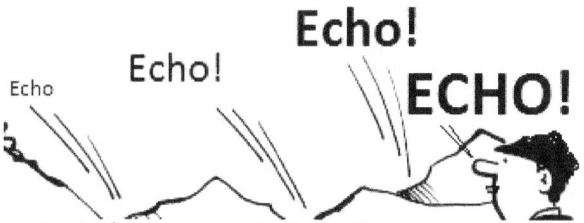

This is the most typical yet extremely limited representation of echo making.

Echoes are sound reflections that return with a certain amount of delay and inevitable loss of intensity, strength, and volume. Studies show that every object and sound has its corresponding echo, but it bounces back so fast that it overlaps the original sound, making it easy to miss in the first place.

Daniel Kish teaches students his version of "flash sonar" by placing a glass panel a few inches from their faces. He then clicks or asks students to make verbal sound emissions. He then moves the glass to and fro. This changes the sound dynamics of the echoes, making it easier to distinguish if the glass is closer or farther. He calls this technique "systemic stimulus differentiation."

On the other hand, some people can physically perceive sound waves when these travel through air. They feel slight changes in air currents (e.g. changes in temperature, or air flow speed,) and they naturally turn their heads or faces to "gather" more information. This technique is referred to as "facial mapping," or "facial pressure."

Finding which technique works best is highly subjective. Some people quickly learn flash sonar by associating sound with distance and space; while others find facial mapping to be more reliable since they have higher tactile sensitivity. The only way to find out is to try both (or other) techniques and see what works for you.

To make the process easier, practice said techniques using a blindfold. (Make sure that the cloth doesn't cover a large portion of your face.) Sighted people's visual cortex often processes sounds and touch, by matching auditory or tactile stimuli with visual input.

In this case though, you are severely limiting visual stimuli. The brain tries to compensate for the "loss," by heightening the remaining senses, and filling in information gaps with stored knowledge. This is the reason why it is essential to learn ambient noises by heart.

Train your listening and echolocation skills at least an hour every day.

According to the research Dr. Winthrop Niles Kellogg, (an American psychologist who spearheaded human echolocation research in 1964,) sighted people who were deprived of visual input (subjects were blindfolded for hours at a time,) learned to create sonar-like imagery from auditory stimuli. They eventually saw "cartoon-like figures," "ornate buildings," and "whitish green marble" when they practiced echolocation. They learned spatial perception (awareness of given environment,) and had accurately described objects placed several meters aware.

Once you have mastered the 4 previous steps, it is highly recommended that you practice listening and echolocation **at least one hour every day**, as it is easy to revert back to visual stimuli dependency.

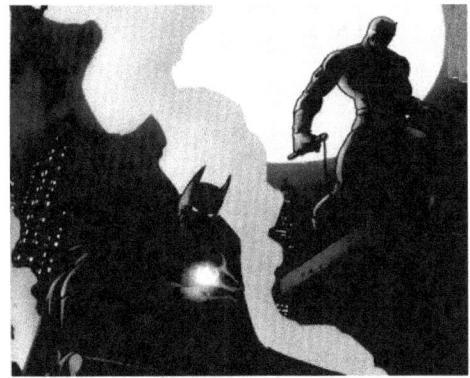

People often associate **Batman** with echolocation, but **Daredevil** has the more superior auditory skills. Image source: www.gibicomicscans.blogspot.com.br

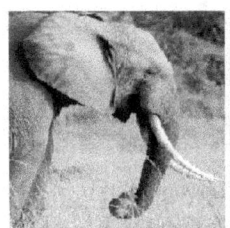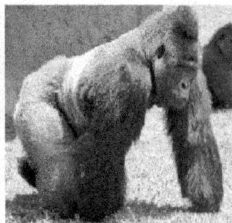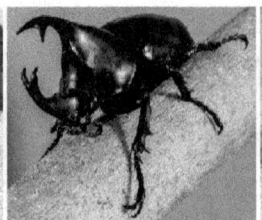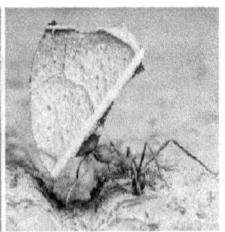

Elephants and gorillas are just two of the strongest land-based animals. In the insect world, rhinoceros beetles' and leaf cutter ants' strength are unsurpassable.
Image Source: www.pixabay.com.

Extreme Feats of Strength

African elephants are known for their brute strength. Adult males can easily transport up to 9,000 kg. / 19,842 lbs. of load in one trip. Silverback gorillas can lift objects up to 2,000 kg. / 4,409 lbs. (approximately ten times their weight) over their heads and hurl it 10 to 12 meters away.

If you measure pound per pound ratio, rhinoceros beetles and leaf cutter ants can lift objects 850 and 50 times their own weight, respectively. That's like an elephant carrying 850 more elephants on its back, or a gorilla hurling five other full-grown gorillas into the air all at once.

There are also numerous people who regularly showcase incredible feats of strength.

In 2016, Asha "Iron Queen" Rani from India hauled a London double decker bus at a distance of five meters using only her hair. Olga Liashchuk from Ukraine crushed three watermelons using only her thighs in just 14.65 seconds. Both of these ladies have multiple world records.

In 2015, Brian Shaw from USA, won the strongest man competition for the 3rd time. His records included: bench press at 238 kg. / 525 lbs., deadlift at 400 kg. / 882 lbs., and squat lift at 360 kilograms / 794 pounds. Igor Zaripov of Russia set his world record that same year when he pulled a bus that weighed 13,713.6 kg. / 30,233 lbs. at a distance of five meters using only his teeth.

But the "average" person can display incredible feats of strength, too.

In January 2016, 19 year old Charlotte Heffelmire (USA,) lifted a burning truck off her father twice. Eric Heffelmire was working under his vehicle when the jack slipped. The gas line ruptured and ignited. 5'6" and 120 lb. Charlotte successfully pulled her father out after two attempts, and then drove the lit truck into the garage to contain the fire. She evacuated her father and her little sister from the premises, and called 911 for help. (Source: www.dailymail.co.uk)

In February 2006, Lydia Angyiou (Canada,) fought off a 700 lb. Polar bear that stalked her 7 year old son as the latter played in the snow. Described as diminutive and lean, the 41 year old woman ended up wrestling with the bear! A neighbor had to shoot the animal four times before it desisted. Angyiou and her son survived the attack. (Source: www.theglobeandmail.com)

When it comes to acquiring super strength, it is not just about gaining muscle or having brute strength. One must also have agility, endurance, and quick reflexes. Having presence of mind is also highly beneficial. Otherwise, you end up with an impressive physique that serves no purpose.

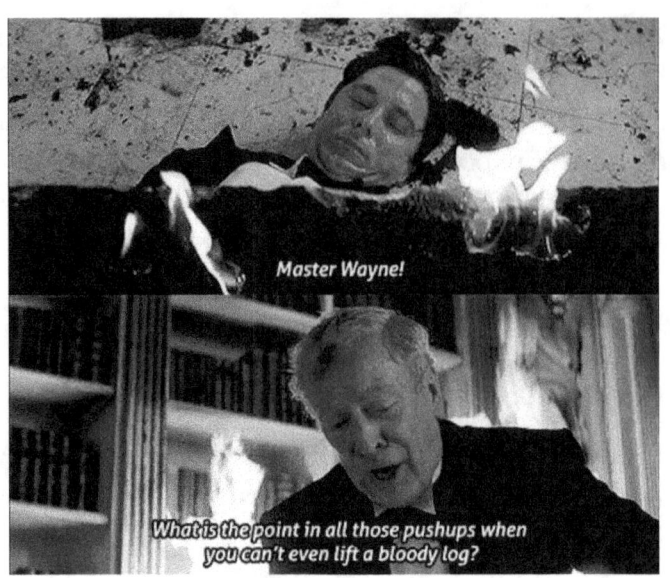
Alfred tells it like it is: "Master Wayne!
What is the point in all those pushups when you can't even lift a bloody log?"
Image source: www.s-media-cache-ako.pinimg.com

But how?

People react differently during a crisis. Some experience surges of adrenaline during critical moments. An unusual amount of hormones and proteins are produced by the body, which are then diverted into bones, muscles, and nerves. This is inexplicably triggered by the adrenal medulla, which is responsible for producing endorphins, dopamine, serotonin, and oxytocin – the four neuro-chemicals associated with happiness.

Some psychologists refer to this condition as "hysterical strength," (positive) or "excited delirium," (negative.)

Research suggests that the effects of hysterical strength and excited delirium are similar to taking dangerous stimulants like amphetamines: a prohibited performance-enhancing drug that increases acceleration, endurance, muscular strength, speed, and stamina.

But there are a few notable differences, such as:

Effects of amphetamine and adrenaline on the human body

	Amphetamine	Adrenaline rush due to:	
		Hysterical strength	Excited delirium
Increased acceleration	Yes	Yes	Yes
Increased endurance	Yes	Yes	Yes
Increased muscular strength	Yes	Yes	Yes
Increased speed	Yes	Yes	Yes
Increased stamina	Yes	Yes	Yes
Increased reflexes	**No**	**Yes**	**No**
Increased brain activity	**No**	**Yes**	**No**
Ability to make life-saving decisions	**No**	**Yes**	**No**
Prolonged effects	Depends on dosage, chronic use, and drug tolerance	No	Depends on person's initial mental state
Permanent damage to brain cells	Yes	No	Depends on person's initial mental state
Permanent damage to the liver	Yes	No	No

Permanent damage to nerve endings	Yes	No	No
Permanent damage to central nervous system	Yes	No	No
Long-time damage to the body	Yes	No	Depends on actions taken during delirium
Delays or inhibits healing	Yes	No	No
Lowers/suppresses immunity	Yes	No	No
Potential carcinogen	Yes	No	No
Anxiety	No	No	Yes
Hallucinations	When chronically abused	No	Yes
Insensitivity to pain	No	No	Yes
Disorientation	No	No	Yes
Speech disturbances/ inability to articulate	No	No	Yes
Elevated body temperature	When chronically abused	No	Yes
Delirium	No	No	Yes
Bizarre/violent behavior	No	No	Yes

Hysterical strength and excited delirium are just a couple of ways on how the human body can achieve super strength. But there are other, more organic, and safer methods of doing so.

Advantages of having super strength

Aside from being able to lift the sofa easily so you can vacuum underneath it, or haul barbells in the gym like these weigh nothing to impress some of the girls, there are a few other benefits of having immense physical power, like:

You can protect yourself, and your family better.
In 2013, Jeff Smith (USA) was pinned under a 3,000 lb. tractor after the vehicle accidentally flipped over. His daughters Hannah (16 years old,) and Haylee (14 years old) just came home from school and were alerted by the family dog's barking. With their combined effort, they managed to tilt the tractor so that their father could wriggle out from underneath. Jeff Smith suffered from a broken wrist, but escaped the ordeal with his life. (Source: www.foxnews.com/us/2013/04/11/)

You can help save lives.
Brittnie Peck from (USA) rescued an infant who was left inside a parked mini-van. Peck saw the distressed child, and broke through the window of the van. The temperature inside was a steaming 97°C (206°F,) which was hot enough to broil the little boy alive. When rescue officers arrived, it was discovered that the year-old infant was left on his own for 45 minutes while his father went into a restaurant. Peck soothed the baby and calmed him down until the paramedics arrived. Police said that if the infant stayed another 5 minutes within, he would've died from asphyxiation, heat stroke, and stress. (Source: www.wbay.com/2016/06/14/woman-rescues-child-from-hot-car)

You can think and react faster than most people.
Delroy Simmonds from Brooklyn, New York, jumped into the tracks of an oncoming subway train to save the life of a 9-month-old boy. The stroller where the infant was strapped in accidentally rolled

into the tracks. Simmonds jumped in and hoisted the boy and stroller to safety. Because of his heroism, he missed an important job interview. According to Simmonds, it as a fatherly instinct as he had two daughters of his own.(Source:http://www.nydailynews.com)

You can set or break world records, if desired.

Many people who build and sculpt their physique often do so in order to enter competitions. Some even aspire to and break or set new world records. Although that is admirable, you can also set a different kind of record – one that saves hundreds, thousands, or millions of lives.

In 1986, a catastrophic accident happened in the Chernobyl nuclear power plant (USSR.) A reactor core was overheating. This would have caused an explosion that would have wiped out both Asian and European continents.

Three brave souls named: Alexei Ananenko, Boris Baranov, and Valeri Bezpalov volunteered to flood and drain the reactor. Then they dropped bags of sand to control the leak. Their physically grueling tasks contained the radiation considerably, and saved millions of lives. (Source: www.storypick.com)

You can remain at the peak of your health for a long time.

This means that your agility, endurance, and stamina are enhanced even at an advanced age. Incredibly, there are a number of elderly folks these days who are fit, trim, and fashionable.

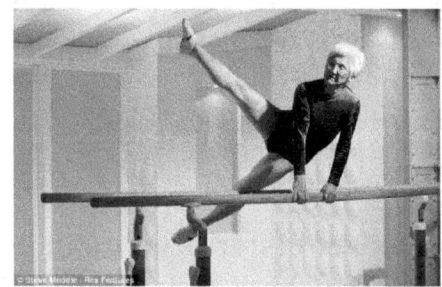

Johanna Quaas, often referred to as Super Gran,
performs her routine on the parallel bars.
Image source: www.dailymail.co.uk

Johanna Quaas, (91 years old) is in the Guinness Book of World Records for being the oldest active gymnast in the world. This diminutive lady from Germany still competes to this day.

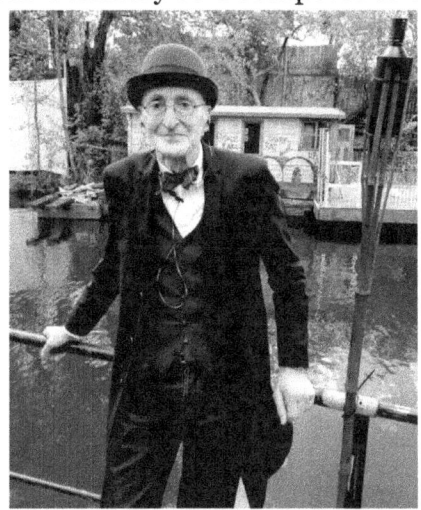

Hipster Grandpa Günther Krabbenhöft is one
fashionable dude.
Image source: www.womendailymagazine.com

Günther Krabbenhöft, also from Germany is an internet sensation. Not only does he look fit and spry, but his fashion sense is on-point as well. His social media accounts has millions of followers.

Basic Guidelines on Power Training

Subscribe to a healthier lifestyle.
Having incredible strength starts with getting fit. Some people might be more naturally gifted with greater physique, but the human body can always benefit more from further conditioning.

Get a clean bill of health from your doctor.
Undergo a complete physical check-up. Ask your doctor how you can improve your health especially if you are going to switch diets, or if you are subscribing to a more rigorous exercise regimen. If you have any underlying medical conditions (e.g. diabetes, heart ailments, liver disorders, etc.) or recently underwent any medical procedure (e.g. chemotherapy, physical therapy, surgery, etc.) ask your doctor how you can safely work without aggravating or compromising your health further.

Subscribe to a better diet.
It doesn't matter what kind of eating regimen you wish to follow. The important thing is that you acquire organic vitamins and minerals from your daily meals. If possible, cut back on processed food items, and unnecessary food supplements.

Add more colors to your diet whenever possible. Green leafy vegetables, and vibrantly colored fruits have loads of digestion-friendly enzymes that aid weight loss. These promote better nutrient absorption, and speed up toxin removal. This benefits digestive and renal systems well.

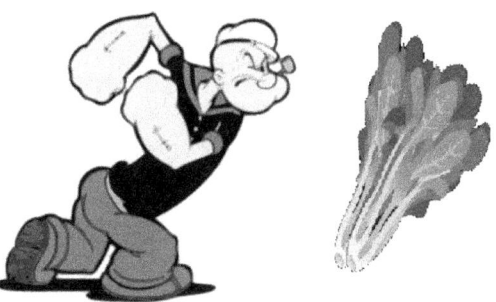

Popeye gains his super strength by regularly eating spinach.
Low in cholesterol and fat, these leafy greens have high amounts of:
antioxidants, calcium, copper, fiber, folate, iron, manganese, niacin,
phosphorus, potassium, protein, thiamine, zinc and Vitamins A, C, E and K.
Image source: www.pixabay.com.

Vegetables and fruits contain antioxidants that speed up cell regeneration and rejuvenation. These improve the health of your hair, nails and skin, which makes you feel and look young. More importantly, a diet high in fresh produce speeds up muscle building, and prevent bones from breaking during rigorous workouts.

You don't have to become a vegetarian or vegan to reap the benefits of consuming fresh fruits and vegetables. Simply adding 1 cup of fresh/raw vegetables (or ½ cup of lightly cooked greens,) and ¼ cup of fresh fruits to your meals will suffice.

With a few rare exceptions (like: brined capers, frozen peas, and olives preserved in oil, etc.) avoid consuming processed fruits and vegetables. Many of these no longer contain usable nutrients, and some are packed with high amounts of salt and sweeteners.

Avoid commercially produced fruit juices and fruit-based sodas, too. These contain food additives, preservatives, and sugar that are detrimental to ones' health.

Shed off unwanted poundage

No one wants to hear that they need to lose weight, but in order to acquire super strength, this step is critical. Muscles can't develop properly if there are generous layers of fat around these.

Fat cells (also called adipose tissues) absorb moisture like sponges. These add considerable weight to bones, which increases the risk of breakage. Excess weight also increases the risk of torn ligaments, muscles, and tendons too, and strains the lower lumbar area that causes chronic back pains.

Cut back on food items, drinks, or practices that are detrimental to your health in general.

These include (but not limited to):

- Chronically being stressed (emotionally, mentally, and physically)
- Constantly worrying, which also leads to undue stress
- Excessive consumption of alcoholic beverages
- Excessive consumption of fat, salt and sweets
- Excessive consumption of coffee and other nerve-stimulating drinks
- Doing hard or recreational drugs
- Not getting enough sleep or rest every day/night
- Physically stressing certain body parts due to laziness (e.g. poor posture stresses the lower lumbar area, carrying all your shopping in one go puts a lot of pressure on digits, joints and tendons, etc.)
- Promiscuity
- Smoking
- Spending too much time in the sun and not using any kind of protection (e.g. caps/hats, dark glasses, sunblock lotion, etc.)
- Spending too much time in any sedentary activity (e.g. sitting on a couch and gossiping, watching TV, etc.)

Start any exercise regimen

Building up your super strength means building up your physique – and you can't really do that if you sit in front of the computer or TV all the time.

Try low-impact cardio workouts first, like: ballroom dancing, cycling, step aerobics, swimming, tai chi, walking, and water aerobics. Exercising for as little as 30 minutes, three times a week easily burns off 3,000 calories – more, if you increase duration, frequency, and intensity.

Exercising on elliptical bikes, rowing machines, or stair masters works too. These don't add undue stress on bones, joints, ligaments and tendons.

If you like being outdoors, try cross-country skiing, hiking, kayaking, rollerblading, rock climbing, and snow shoeing. Golf can also be considered as a low impact workout if you walk the entire course.

Pilates, strength training, total body resistance exercises, and yoga burn off the most calories – approximately 5,000 to 7,000 calories for an hour long, twice a week session.

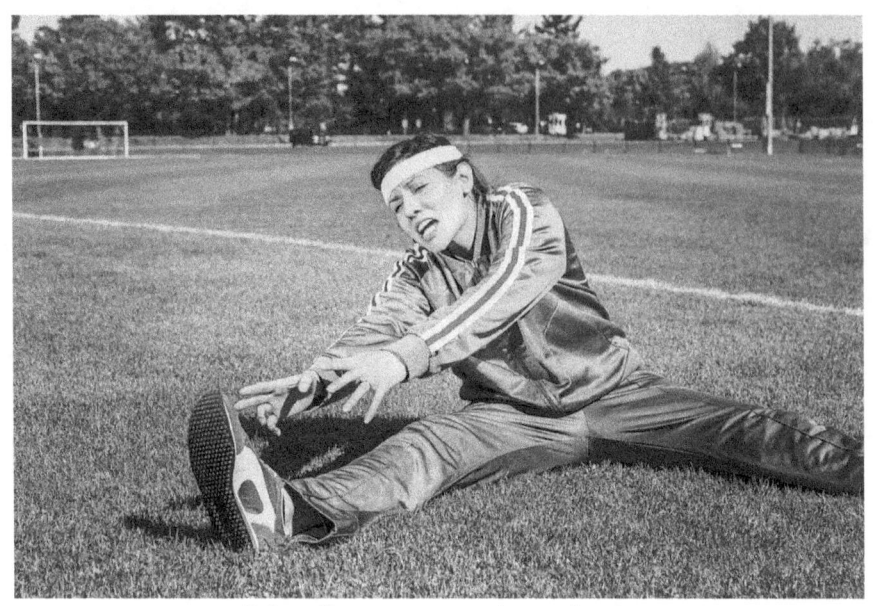
Subscribe to any exercise regimen.
Acquiring super powers entails more than just sitting in front of the computer or TV all day.
Image source: www.pixabay.com.

Start your strength training, preferably under the supervision of a qualified trainer.
After shedding off unwanted poundage, your next step is to develop your core muscles. These are responsible for building up intense strength, particularly in the long muscles of the arms and legs, in the midsection, and in the back.

Although you can always do strength training on your own, having a personal trainer at your side can speed up the process quickly and safely.

Become more agile
Being agile means that you can act or move quickly. Having super strength doesn't mean that you should only spend your days

working out and lifting heavy objects. You should be fast and flexible too.

Iran. A viral video showed an unnamed 14 year old boy as he caught a toddler who fell from a height. The young man was first seen looking up, as if he already spotted trouble. He walked on, but then retraced his steps. He dropped the bag of chips he was holding, and caught a toddler who fell off an escalator railing. Although both of them took a tumble, the child was saved from certain death or serious injury. The video was first uploaded in November 2015 and has since reached over 1 million views. (Source: www.express.co.uk)

Here are some exercises that can help you become agile.

Rope skipping, moderate speed, 15 minutes a day, every day. Aside from burning off 16 to 20 calories per minute, rope skipping on the balls of your feet helps improve your balance considerably. Your body automatically makes muscular adjustments so that you remain upright all throughout. This realigns your spine and improves your posture.

Rope skipping adds flexibility to your legs' ligaments and tendons, and the constant bouncing increases bone density.

Swimming (breast stroke) and/or water aerobics, slow to moderate intensity or speed, 30 minutes, two times a week. These exercises off around 400 to 800 calories (depending on intensity) in just 30 minutes. These trains the long muscles of the arms and legs better than Pilates or yoga.

Moving through water provides enough resistance to exert muscular strength, but without straining ligaments and tendons in elbows, knees, spine, and shoulders. This is a great cardiovascular workout too, as the heart tends to beat a little faster (due to buoyancy) when the body is submerged in water.

Best of all, recent studies show that regularly exercising in the water improves sleep by 50% to 75%.

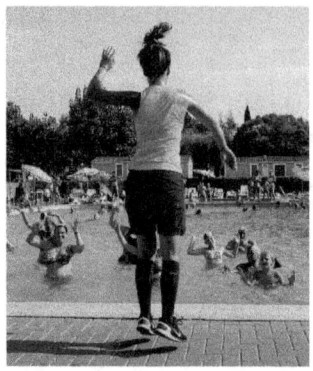

Aquaman approves of all forms of water exercises.
Image source: www.pixabay.com

Trampoline exercises/jumping, moderate speed, 20 minutes a day, three to four times a week. Similar to rope skipping, rebounding on the trampoline increase flexibility, realigns the spine, and burns off about 20 to 25 calories per minute. It improves the cardiovascular system, as a person naturally hold his/her breath just before the jumping, and exhale when going down. Higher jumps mean deeper and longer breaths, and the body is consuming more oxygen.

This provides mental clarity and triggers production of endorphins, dopamine, serotonin, and oxytocin. This is the reason why people experience euphoric feelings during high jumps.

Build up more endurance and stamina. Find your motivation.
The word "endurance" is sometimes confused with "perseverance" but the latter is only one aspect of the former. Human endurance is the willpower to bear hardship and pain, despite hunger, fatigue,

stress, or other adverse conditions. It is that force that pushes the person to survive or persevere in order to meet certain aspirations or goals. In many cases, endurance means pushing your body and spirit to their breaking point – and live to tell the tale.

Although endurance (via physical training) can be taught, it's really a case of mind over matter. When all things fail, when nothing seems to go right, when everything seems desperately hopeless, what will push you to go further?

This is where motivation takes hold.

Some survivors of horrific accidents claim that their desire to be with their loved ones motivate them to push through. Others are propelled by the thought of surviving in order to set things right with family and friends. Others are compelled by promises they made, or perceived rewards afterwards.

17 year old Juliane Koepcke (from Germany) survived a plane crash that claimed the life of her mother and 90 others. On Christmas eve of 1971, the young girl tumbled out of the broken plane, and through a thick canopy of trees while still strapped to her seat. She had a broken collar bone, ruptured ligament in her knee, and deep cuts on her arms and legs. She staggered alone in a Peruvian rainforest (where the plane crashed) for 10 days. She eventually found a group of locals who fed her, treated her maggot-infested wounds, and brought her back to civilization. (Source: www.bbc.com/news/magazine)

In 2011, Richard Moyer (USA) got up as usual at 3 a.m. to let their dog out. When their pet came back in, it was closely followed by a fully grown black bear. It attacked Richard. His wife Angela woke up from the commotion. She distracted the bear into letting go of her husband, but the beast turned on her. It clamped down hard on her arm, and dragged her outside. Richard jumped on the bear, but got bit in the head. Inexplicably, the animal stopped its vicious attack and walked away. Angela suffered from a cracked vertebra, and multiple bites all over. Richard suffered from multiple bites and deep scratches. He also had puncture wounds at the back of his head where he got bit. (Source: www.edition.cnn.com)

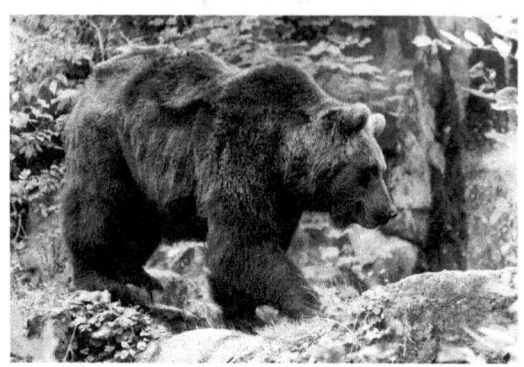

Black bears are powerful animals. A single swipe
from their 9-inch claws can easily disembowel a man.
They also have a 64 bite force quotient
- enough to crush in a man's head.
Image source: www.pixabay.com.

The couples' motivation to keep fighting was their 10 year old son, who was asleep in the upstairs bedroom at that time. The last thing they wanted was to leave their little boy in the hands of the bear.

Bravery and courage, and the need to act.

Ever had one of those moments when you felt the need to do something during potentially dangerous situations, but people held you back "for your own safety?"

This is one of the biggest reasons why a lot of people hesitate to take action or don't take action at all during crucial moments. A person's sense of self-preservation is often combined with the community's collective need to stay out of danger. Others simply stand aside or walk away because they don't have the courage to stand up to adversity, or they simply don't know how to act in the face of danger.

Just to clarify matters: having bravery and courage is not about doing reckless things, or showing off fearlessness by doing dangerous stunts. It's certainly not about posting scary escapades into abandoned building on the Internet, or performing potentially spine-shattering tricks in front of the camera. In most cases these are nothing more than heedless actions taken with the intent to impress others.

A man trying to beat a moving train by jumping the tracks, and getting killed in the process is neither brave nor courageous. But a man who jumps into the path of an incoming subway train to save the life of a child, and then walks away without recognition or thanks shows not only bravery and courage, but great humility as well.

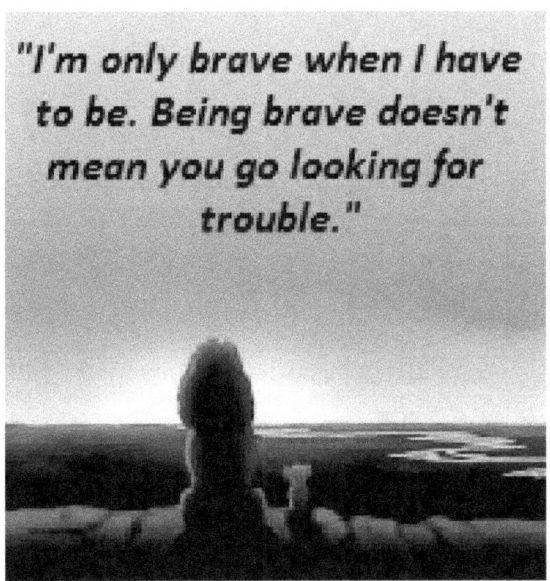

King Mufasa schools his son about bravery. (Lion King)
Image source: www.pixabay.com

According to Merriam-Webster dictionary (www.merriam-webster.com,) bravery is "acquired or inherent quality that allows a person to do dangerous or terrifying actions without feeling or showing fear. Having courage is "the ability to act knowing that conditions are difficult, dangerous, or potentially life-threatening in the first place."

There are some people who seem to be inherently brave/courageous, but this ability can also be acquired through study and practice.

For example: a man jumps into a frozen lake to save the life of a drowning woman. He does this with confidence because he knows he is a good swimmer. He had also swum in the same frozen lake before, and that at one point learned basic first aid.

Helping save lives is always considered as an impressive showcase of strength, bravery, and courage in the face of danger.

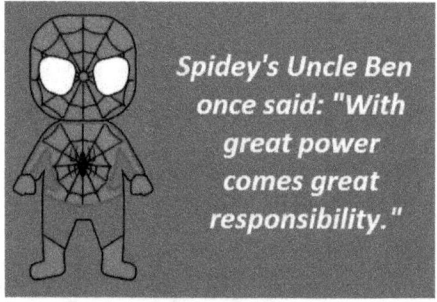

Image source: www.pixabay.com

Few tips on how you can potentially help others at a time of need.

Learn first aid measures.
Basic first aid measures like: CPR and Heimlich maneuver can save lives, especially if you are miles away from the nearest clinic or hospital. During medical intervention, every second matters. When the body is deprived of oxygen, permanent brain damage, spinal damage, and even death can occur within minutes. It is essential that you keep the person in need stable and breathing until trained rescuers arrive.

Few examples of basic first aid measures include:

CPR. Cardiopulmonary resuscitation is often performed on someone whose breathing or heartbeat has stopped. This may be due to drowning, electric shock, heart attack, or lightning strike, etc.

Heimlich maneuver or abdominal thrusts. This is performed on choking victims. Pressure is applied on the bottom of the diaphragm, which compresses the lungs. When done correctly, the air from the lungs move with such force that any obstruction in the trachea is expelled.

Managing bleeding and physical shock. A person's life is in danger if he/she loses a lot of blood in a short amount of time. Pressure should be applied on afflicted parts to staunch the flow of blood. Shock and trauma follow quickly if a bleeding person's blood pressure is not stabilized in time.

Managing broken bones, dislocated limbs, fractures, etc. These conditions are extremely painful, and may lead to blood loss,

loss of limb(s,) permanent paralysis due to spinal damage, shock, unconsciousness, and even death.

Managing burns. The most common first aid measure for first and second degree burns is to apply cold to the afflicted body part. This stops the heat from spreading and damaging more tissues. However, third degree burns are more critical. Afflicted body parts should be wrapped gently in damp cloth to prevent infection.

Learning a few advance life-saving measures won't hurt as well. These include: (but are not limited to)
Delivering a baby during emergency situations.

Helping someone who has alcohol, drug or substance poisoning.

Helping someone who is experiencing blood poisoning (due to unstable blood sugar-insulin levels, chemical and gas poisoning, or food and water-borne contaminants.)

Helping someone who may potentially have spinal injury.

Helping someone who suffered from head injury.

Managing frostbite or heat stroke.

Resuscitating newborns and infants.

Stabilizing people who may be suffering from epilepsy, heart attacks, or stroke.

Treating animal bites or effects of animal attacks.

Treating life-threatening symptoms of allergies, like anaphylactic shock from bee stings, latex, peanuts, penicillin, and shellfish, etc.

There are community centers or local health facilities who regularly offer first aid courses for free. They provide hands-on training exercises, and can introduce you to other life-saving tools and organizations. If these are not available in your area, you can always look up online tutorials, and practice these life saving measures on your own.

If the occasion calls for it, you may need to use your super strength to lift or transport a person out of immediate danger. You can always carry someone in your arms, or have him/her rid piggyback.

You can also try the fireman's carry – a technique by which the person you are transporting is draped across your shoulder. This enables you to move quickly despite the additional weight because you can see what's right in front of you.

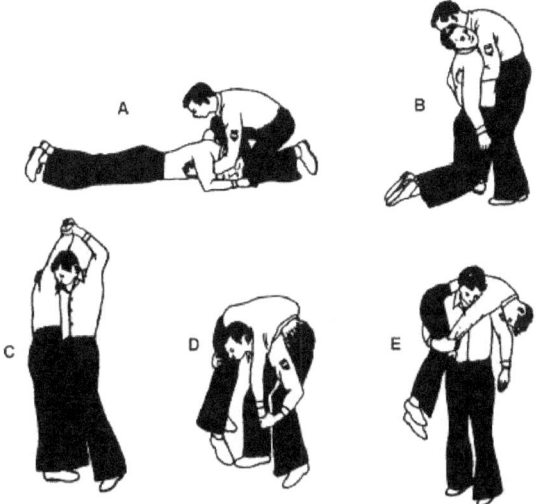

A diagram showing how to perform the fireman's carry on an unconscious person. Image source: www.artofmanliness.com/2011/03/29/how-to-perform-the-firemans-carry/

Learn how to swim. Drowning is a common cause of accidental death in children under the age of 15. More often than not, any intervention from surrounding people can help save their lives, like: cradling the child so his/her head is above water, reaching out and physically pulling the child out of the water, or even just providing an arm, a floatation device, or a safety ring to hold on to.

Unfortunately, many people refuse to go into the water because they can't swim, or they don't think they're strong enough to rescue drowning victims.

Swimming should in your skill arsenal. Not only will this potentially save lives, but it can also save yours.

Keep a watchful eye at all times. Be aware of your surroundings so that you can sense if trouble is brewing. Prevention is always preferable, of course, but learning some defensive moves can help you feel safe too.

Practice life-saving scenarios with friends and family. One of the primary reasons why some people don't hesitate to help is that they know precisely what to do in particular situations. They may have had prior experience, or have previously learned ways on how to react to certain dangers.

Whenever possible, create and practice safety drills in your home or community. This may include: (but not limited to)
How to quickly and safely evacuating your house or building when fire or earthquakes occur.

Teaching family members non-verbal codes (e.g. clapping, finger snaps, switching the lights on or off, whistling, etc.) that would signify a call for help, if or when there are intruders in the house.

Teaching your kids or younger siblings/relatives what to do during dangerous or emergency situations, e.g. what to say to a 911 dispatcher, making them memorize loved ones' or neighbors' phone numbers who can help, etc.

Final Thoughts

There are many superpowers in the comic universe like: the ability to fly, heal from all injuries, or walk through walls. Some powers are gained through study and practice, like: casting magic spells or becoming an expert in hand-to-hand combat.

The same is true when it comes to developing your own skills and superpowers. This book contains basic information on most common powers that many people are actually using in real life, namely: echolocation and impressive feats of strength.

Hopefully, this book has given you some basic tips on how to unlock your unique powers through foresight, study and training.

Good luck to you in your journey!